Fasting – 7 Steps to Health and Happiness

Lose Weight and Feel Great with Fasting

Dr. Michelle Danville

Disclaimer:

Table of Contents

Introduction

In the 2016 report of the National Center for Health Statistics (NCHS), 70.2% or 2 in 3 adults are overweight and obese. Breaking the figures by gender, the report shows overweight men at 38.7% and 26.5% women. Going to the statistics on obesity, the percentage for obese women is higher at 40% than the men (35 %.)

The same report claims an increasing trend in the prevalence of overweight and obesity among adults. From 2005 to 2014, the increase in obesity is significant in women with no significant increase for men.

One is overweight or obese if the weight is above the normal weight appropriate to one's height. Being overweight or obese exposes you to health problems such as type 2 diabetes, joint problems, gallstones, and high blood pressure. Studies show a close association between obesity and certain types of cancer, osteoarthritis, sleep apnea and other non communicable diseases.

Living in today's modern society, the increase in overweight and obese adults is not surprising. While gene contributes to obesity, another major contributing factor is one's lifestyle evident in your eating habits, a sedentary life aided by technology, and sleeping habits.

Many women find fasting as the answer to fight obesity. But, there are many reports from women experiencing discomforts when fasting. The failure to lose weight can be attributed to several factors, to name a few:

- Not clear with what fasting is
- Misinformation or wrong information about fasting
- Lack of medical understanding about fasting

Today, the number of fasting methods offered by individuals claiming to be experts, associations, and organizations could be confusing. Most fasting methods promoted seldom consider the many differences between men and women. Differences, if recognized and acknowledged, could spell success for women who fast.

If you plan to go on fasting for health and longer life, the questions to ask are: How to choose a fasting plan that works for you, and how do you start fasting?

Chapter 1

Fasting Throughout History

Do you know how the word "breakfast" came about?

We know that breakfast is the first meal you take after a night's sleep. However, the term is revealing as it means breaking a fast of the night before, which you did when you slept.

From the term, you get a glimpse of fasting as a natural biological tendency of man to give the body rest, balance, and save energy after a day's work or during critical times. For instance, you lose your appetite in times of stress or when you feel sick. Fasting is a natural healing therapy used by the early people, which continued to the present.

Fasting in primitive people

Fasting has older roots in the primitive times, with dietary restrictions referred to by the primitive people as 'taboo.' Considered taboos are certain vegetables and animals, and eating of specific food during particular days of the year. These people practice dietary restrictions for health and safety reasons. However, artifacts exist that depict not only restrictions but fasting or abstinence from food.

Fasting for the primitive people was motivated by:

Special rituals. Primitive people fasts during important events, like initiating their youth into adulthood. Fasting could last from 24 hours to days. They also fast before the consumption of a new harvest, before engaging in a tribal war, and before hunting.

Purification. Purification of the body is similar to the modern-day concept; the difference lies in the purpose. For the primitive people, purifying the body is to prepare it for a purpose, to give thanks, and to offer to or receive a reward from a deity. The idea of fasting is to bring the body to an improved state deserving of a deity's reward.

Mysticism. Shamans and ancient priests fast to appease the anger of vengeful spirits or their deities. Primitive hunters fast to make themselves deserving of their quarry. And, the farmers fast for the earth and weather spirits to favor bountiful harvest.

Fasting for the Early Greeks

The early Greek people practiced fasting for health and therapeutic purposes. The Greek philosophers, such as Pythagoras, Hippocrates, Plato, Aristotle, Socrates, and Galen advocated fasting as a natural health remedy.

Paracelsus cited fasting as the 'physician within' referring to the internal mechanisms that protect the body system. Hippocrates, known as the father of medicine, prescribed the use of fasting and recommended taking the apple cider vinegar. Plutarch supported fasting as a natural remedy instead of medicine. Pythagoras went on 40 days fast with water to sustain him, believing that abstaining from food results to enhanced creativity and mental perception.

The early Greeks believed in the natural healing capacity of man, much like nature, which is almost instinctual. For the early Greeks, fasting has a rejuvenating and revitalizing power.

Fasting in religion

Fasting played a spiritual role in ancient religions; to this day, it remains a part of major religions worldwide. Jesus Christ, the prophet Muhammed, and Buddha shared the belief in fasting for health purposes and for the benefits it gives to the body. Fasting was also practiced spiritually for purification.

Traces of primitive rites of fasting can be seen in ancient and modern-day religious practices:

- The symbolic use of the unleavened bread by the Jews during the Passover traces back to the primitive rites
- Muslims' observance of fast by day and not after dark during Ramadan symbolizes penitence which is reminiscent of ancient practices
- Early Christians' fasting is a symbolism for penitence and purification, which the primitive people did in preparation for offering their purified selves to a deity. The practice of fasting today is also done as a preparation before receiving the sacraments of Holy Communion, baptism, and ordination of priests.

Modern-day Fasting

Today, the original concept of fasting became modified and complicated. Fasting became complicated with the addition of other items, like juices instead of water, fruits, and other nutritious food. Technically, the modern concept of restrictions will fall under 'diets' which many refer to as 'cleansing' diets or 'detox diets.'

Regardless of the term used to signify fasting, there is hope for its health and therapeutic use.

Some healers and physicians with spiritual and holistic orientation recommend the use of fasting for health purposes. Conventional medicine does not fully recognize fasting as a natural health remedy. However, the idea of the body-mind connection is gradually taking hold in the field of modern-day medicine.

Physicians today are willing to accept fasting, not to interfere with the practice, but to build up the body's healing mechanisms. With this acceptance, fasting may recover its original concept as a self-healing mechanism of the body.

Currently, many researchers conduct studies on the unseen energy that naturally moves the body towards health and balance. Some physicians believe the field of medicine will encompass the study of the body's energy patterns. Knowledge obtained from these studies can enhance the energy patterns for the man's health and well-being.

The purpose of fasting varies, and the benefits you get when you fast are many. Physically, fasting is a natural resting period during which time the body eliminates the stored waste material so greater healing can happen. Spiritually, religious people believe that fasting provides the opportunity for clarity and insights that can lead to stronger faith and understanding.

Chapter 2

Wrong Information Turned Right

Fasting is gaining in popularity, and many women are getting into some form of diet and exercise regimens to lose weight or for other purposes. Many of these regimens have scientific bases, though distortion of facts occurred through time.

In the desire to capture a share of the weight loss industry, the scientific facts become distorted or omitted for the sake of revenues, benefits exaggerated, and the risks involved downplayed.

Women, in particular, should be wary of the different diets and exercises promoted. Different diet plans give out information which may not be correct. In time, the misinformation on fasting becomes myths, which adds to your confusion when choosing the right approach that works for you.

Eating breakfast makes you fat.

Many people believe that missing breakfast will lead to excessive hunger and craving resulting to gain in weight. Studies on the relationship of skipping breakfast to obesity claim a link between the two variables. However, the gain in weight happens to those skippers who are not health-conscious.

A 2014 study clarified the concern on skipping breakfast with its conclusion that skipping breakfast does not make a difference in weight loss. What the study means is that whether you eat or skip breakfast will not make a difference in your weight.

It may happen that skipping or eating breakfasts have different outcomes on different individuals. For instance, some studies report of children and youth who eat breakfast perform better in school. Other studies also show that there are people who eat breakfast who succeed in their weight loss program in the long run.

Truth: The bottom line is that having breakfast can benefit people, but it is not essential.

Frequent eating can boost your metabolism

A popular belief about fasting is that eating more meals increases your metabolic rate allowing your body to burn more calories.

There is a degree of truth in this belief since the body spends energy digesting and assimilating the nutrients in the food you consume. This process is called the Thermic Effect of Food (TEF.) But, on average, the TEF is only about 10% of the total calorie intake.

Truth: The important thing in consumption is not the frequency of meals. What are necessary are the amount of calorie in the food and the breakdown of macronutrients that make a significant difference to your body.

Frequent eating helps reduce hunger

It is the belief of many that eating between meals prevents excessive hunger and food craving. Studies done on this concern show mixed results.

Some of these studies report a reduction in hunger with more meals, others claim there is no significant difference in the frequency of meals, and still others with contradicting results report having more meals tend to increase the hunger level.

Truth: What these conflicting studies reveal is that the effects of meal frequency to hunger drive would depend on the individuals concerned. There is, however, no evidence to show that eating more often eliminates hunger and reduce calorie intake.

Frequency of small meals helps you lose weight

The frequency of meals does not boost your metabolism or reduce the craving for food. If meal frequency does not affect your metabolism and food craving, then, it has no bearing on weight loss. Many studies support the conclusion on the impact of meal frequency on weight.

Truth: It does not matter how often you eat or how many meals you take. What matters is the amount of calorie and nutrient you consume.

Our brain needs glucose to function

We often hear people say that our brain needs glucose for its proper functioning. This information is incorrect as our brains use ketones as the source of fuel during starvation, like when you are fasting. Ketones are byproducts of the body which break down fat to use as energy when glucose is not available.

The use of fat is our body's way of saving food energy for the long-term, while glucose is for the short-term. Therefore, when the short-term glucose deplete, the body turns to stored fat for energy fuel. This condition happens when you fast and abstain from food.

Truth: Traditional nutrition says that glucose is the primary source of energy for the body.

When the glucose deplete, the cells switch to fat as a source of energy. The current researches show that fat, as a source of energy, is healthier than glucose and more sustainable.

You put your body on starvation mode when fasting

The starvation mode, again, is wrong information fed to us as a child or as we grow up. When we skip a meal as a child, our parents scare us with the threat of our body shutting down, meaning, a decrease in our metabolism.

But, what about the primitive people who had to hunt for food. A day without food would have weakened the hunters. Going for days without food would make their survival impossible.

What happens when you eat less food is that your energy intake goes down. However, the amount of energy you spend also goes down. At this point, your body switches to stored fat as the source of energy. With the stored fat as energy, you increase the availability of food and increase the level of energy expenditure.

Truth: Studies show that short-term fasting increases our metabolic rate. The increase in metabolism is due to the increase in blood levels which drive the fat cells to break down fat to stimulate metabolism.

You are likely to hear repeated and persistent concerns on overeating, gaining excess weight, food cravings, and starving when fasting.

Remember that fasting is a natural biological way of healing and restoring our body to health. It is a sure and safe way to rid the body of toxic overload to restore the body to health. With a period of abstaining from food, light eating, and quality rest you allow nature to eliminate the toxins in your body.

It is the wrong information on fasting that gets in the way of correct fasting. The science is clear about the effects and benefits of fasting. The myths are but falsehoods wrapped around fasting.

Chapter 3

Healthy Fats for Physical Rejuvenation

Correcting the misinformation on fasting allows you to view it in a new perspective. You begin to realize that fasting, with healthy eating and a healthy lifestyle can help regain your health, rejuvenate your body, and bring back your strength.

Healthy eating means eating food rich in the nutrients you need to maintain a healthy body. These nutrients are carbohydrates, protein, vitamins, minerals, and fat.

As a youth, we were trained to avoid eating fats, believing that food high in fat leads to excess weight and various diseases. When a friend or a doctor tells us to eat food high in fat, our look is one of surprise.

Healthy Fats

Healthy fats are unsaturated fats which could either be monounsaturated or polyunsaturated fats. Unsaturated fats are healthy as they help reduce LDL cholesterol which clogs your arteries. Unsaturated fats regulate insulin and the blood sugar levels, reducing the risk of type 2 diabetes.

Of the two types of unsaturated fats, monounsaturated fat is the healthiest as it is anti-inflammatory, prevents cardiovascular disease, and full of healthy nutrients. Polyunsaturated fats help in brain functions and cell growth.

Healthy Food rich in monounsaturated and polyunsaturated fats

1) *Avocados*. While most fruits are rich in carbohydrates, avocados are rich in fats. Avocados contain 77% fat higher than that found in animal foods. The fruit's main fatty acid is the

monounsaturated fat, referred to as oleic acid, and provides other various health benefits.

Further, avocados contain potassium which is 40% higher than bananas which have high potassium content. This fruit also contains 160 grams of calories, 2 grams of protein, and 9 grams of carbohydrates. However, out of the 9 grams of carbs in avocados, 7 grams are fiber, making this fruit a low-carb diet with 2 grams of net carb.

Though high in fats, people who eat avocado weigh less and show less belly fat compared to people who don't.

2) *Cheese*. Cheese is highly nutritious, given that a slice of cheese is equivalent to a cup of milk. From milk you get calcium, phosphorus, Vitamin B12, protein and selenium. The protein you get from cheese is equivalent to a glass of milk.

Including cheese in your diet meal reduces the risk of type 2 diabetes.

3) *Dark Chocolate*. The incredibly tasty dark chocolate is rich in fat at 65% of calories. It contains 11% fiber and 50% recommended daily allowance (RDA) for magnesium, iron, manganese, and copper. It is high in antioxidants with potent biological activity that lowers blood pressure.

A study reports that people who eat dark chocolate often show improved cardiovascular health than those who don't.

4) *Whole eggs*. Traditionally, whole eggs are considered unhealthy because of the yolks which contain high cholesterol and fat. Recent studies, however, show that an egg contains 212 mg of cholesterol which is equal to 71% of recommended daily consumption, and 62% fat of the calories.

Whole egg is a nutrient dense food which is rich in vitamins and minerals. You can find in eggs a small percent of each nutrient we need.

Other benefits we get from whole eggs:

- Antioxidants that protect the eyes
- Plenty of choline, a nutrient for the brain
- High in protein
- Important for weight loss

If you are adverse to eating eggs because of the yolk, the truth is, you find the nutrients in it.

5) *Fatty Fish*. Fatty fish is good for the health, like salmon, mackerel, trout, herring, and sardines. Fatty fishes are nutritious as they are rich in omega 3 necessary for the optimal functioning of the heart and the brain. Oily fish is a good source of high-quality protein, iodine, and minerals.
People who consume fish prove to be healthier and with a low risk factor for heart disease, dementia, and depression. If you prefer substitutes for fish, you can use cod fish liver oil. This oil contains omega 3 and plenty of Vitamin D.

6) *Nuts*. Nuts are rich in fiber and healthy fats and a rich source of protein. You also find in nuts a high content of

Vitamin E and magnesium. People who eat nuts are healthier and have a lower risk for obesity, heart disease, and type 2 diabetes. Examples of these nuts are walnuts, almonds, and macadamia nuts.

7) *Chia Seeds*. Most people do not see chia seeds as having fats. Contrary to this view, 28 grams of chia seed is equal to 9 grams of fat. Since this seed is fibrous, most calories in this seed come from fat. What makes this seed an excellent source of high-fat plant food is the 80% fat of calories it contains.

Other benefits from chia seeds:
- High in nutrients but low in calories
- Rich in antioxidants. Antioxidants counter the growth of free radicals which damage the molecules in your cells that leads to aging and diseases.
- High in quality protein
- High in important bone nutrients
- Weight loss friendly

8) *Extra Virgin Olive Oil.* Perhaps, no one would argue against extra virgin olive oil as one of the healthiest fats. This oil is a traditional fat used as dietary staple by

most healthy people. It contains fatty acids and antioxidants that have powerful health benefits, one of which is its ability to reduce the risk of heart disease.

A 100 gram of olive oil contains the following nutrients:
- Monounsaturated fats at 73%
- Saturated fat at 13.8%
- Omega 6, 9.7%
- Omega 3, 0.76%
- Vitamin E, 72% of the RDA
- Vitamin K, 75% of the RDA

9) *Lean grass-fed pork and beef.* Contrary to popular belief that steak is high in fat, a steak chosen from a lean cut contains 5 grams of fat and less than 2 grams of saturated fat in each 3-oz of serving. Further, lean meat is a good source of protein, zinc, and iron all of which are good nutrients for active women.

Lean grass-fed beef contains conjugated linoleic acid (CLA) which is a powerful polyunsaturated fatty acid that fights cancer, is weight loss friendly, and builds muscle.

What you gain from eating lean grass-fed beef and pork:
- Fights cancer
- Reduces the risk of heart disease
- Helps maintain a healthy level of blood sugar

Fasting may not be an absolute cure, but healthy eating and living can reverse the errors we made that led to the breakdown of our health.

Chapter 4

Why Fast and What Fasting do to the organs and mind functions

Recently, we see a revival of interest in fasting. The practice of fasting existed in the ancient times, and since then, the concept and reasons why people fast has evolved.

From the primitive time to the present, fasting had been used for medical or therapeutic purposes, religious rites (*for purification*), and political purposes (*sign of protest*.)

The modern concept modified the meaning of the traditional fasting. The original concept of fasting is absolute abstention from food for a day or more with only water to sustain the body. Today, a person who fasts can take other items like juices, fruits, and specific food.

But, what happens to our body when we fast?

Autophagy and Fasting

When we fast, we abstain from food. The abstention lasts for a day or longer, but the effect is the same. We voluntarily deprive or starve ourselves of food for a purpose. However, by fasting, we activate the natural protective mechanism in our body, called autophagy. Autophagy benefits us through the maintenance of our health and the prevention of diseases.

Autophagy comes from a Greek word auto (self), and phagein (to eat) which means to eat one's self. Taken literally, to eat one's self sounds scary. But, this literal translation describes what happens when it does its work.

Autophagy is a mechanism which recycles the organic materials in our cells. Cells grow old, and when this happens, autophagy destroys the old cells and replaces it with new ones to restore homeostasis in our system.

The Importance of autophagy to us

Starvation induces autophagy that leads to the breakdown of organic molecules into amino acids. Autophagy has the potential for self-destruction. Therefore, to prevent self-destruction, autophagy produces a feedback loop. The feedback loop serves as a self-regulatory process that prevents excess self-destruction of autophagy.

Autophagy is necessary for the proper functioning of our cells. We see the importance of autophagy through the role it plays in its different functions:

- *Response to starvation*. Starvation occurs when nutrients and growth factor in the cell are insufficient. The deficiency in nutrients activates autophagy to upregulate. It is necessary for our cells to have a consistent protein synthesis and metabolic rate. And, for our cells to function, autophagy recycles the unnecessary material to produce the amino acids. The amino acids are crucial for protein synthesis to occur. In effect, autophagy supplies the cells temporarily with emergency amino acids during starvation.

- *Cell death.* Just as the maintenance of cell health is important, cell death is of equal necessity for the cells to function properly. When cells are no longer necessary, they die through an intracellular death program where the cells self-destruct in a regulated way. The process of regulated self-destruction is called programmed cell death or apoptosis.

  Cell death is a crucial function in embryonic development. When a cell self-destructs, the death triggers the proteins to produce amino acids necessary for cell survival, which in turn, produce enzymes.

  For instance, in the womb, the fingers and toes of fetus are connected in a web-like form. Apoptosis breaks the web and separates the fingers and toes.

- *Disease mitigation.* This function tops the list of autophagy's importance in the prevention of diseases and illnesses. The role of autophagy in the prevention of diseases is to destroy cells infected with virus and bacteria. It also serves as a protective shield by engulfing the cell, thereby preventing the cell from being infected by foreign bodies.

  Two diseases which autophagy can potentially reverse are encephalopathy and Alzheimer. These two diseases are associated with an increase in damaged protein and other organic materials.

The health benefits we get from autophagy

We cannot discount autophagy's critical role in the maintenance of good health, and in the prevention of non-communicable diseases. Researches on autophagy show that it can reverse the damage to cells caused by oxidative stress. An example of a disease where autophagy can prevent or reverse damaged cell is leukemia.

Other health benefits we get from autophagy through fasting:

- Improved health of brain and cognition.

  A set of metabolic process is essential for maintaining a healthy and functioning brain; this process is triggered by fasting. Fasting contributes to the increase in neurotropic factors essential for the survival, growth, and division of cells. The results of this process show through:

  - Enhanced learning
  - Increased cognitive energy
  - Reduced inflammation in the brain

- Slowing and reversing aging.

  We can view aging as the slow death or dysfunction of cells. Aging happens with the accumulation of damaged proteins and organelles in our cells. When we fast, we activate autophagy which reverses the aging process by removing the damaged cells.

- Improved body composition.

Body composition is the function of our hormonal state. Insulin sensitivity increases during fasting, which in turn, increases adiponectin levels. Insulin and adiponectin are the key hormonal factors that determine if fats are used for energy or if calorie intake is first stored for future use. You experience a calorie deficit while fasting. Your cells get fed by stored fats. And, this hormonal state continues well after fasting.

- Improved digestion.

During fasting, your gastrointestinal tract relaxes which has the effect of reducing intestinal inflammation and improved contraction of digestive muscles. This 'rest period' results to the improvement of nutrient absorption and better bowel movement.

- Cardiovascular health.

Fasting has a positive impact on cardiovascular health. It reduces heart rate and blood pressure during this resting period while increasing the parasympathetic tone (a critical indicator of cardiovascular health.) Another health impact of fasting and autophagy is the improved resilience of the cardiovascular system when in stress.

- Cancer prevention and treatment

    Fasting acts much like the chemotherapy treatment of cancer patients in delaying the growth of tumors. However, while researches show the potential of autophagy to reverse cancer, this is an underutilized tool in cancer treatment.

The myths that surround fasting tend to stop a person from fasting. We usually look at the physical manifestations of fasting like starvation and the discomforts brought by diet change. What escape us are the changes and processes that goes on inside one's body while on fast and the benefits we derive from these changes.

These benefits are significant and are more than enough reasons for us to fast.

Chapter 5

Recovery from Diseases

The past is a trove of treasure when it comes to health. Most of the cures used in modern and alternative medical practices today have their roots from the past.

One health case in point is fasting. The benefits derived from fasting may have been one of the reasons for the revival of interest for it. There is no definite point in time that we can trace the beginnings of fasting. Though, we can safely say our hunter ancestors fast when they hunt their quarry for food. They go without food for days (forced fasting in their case, contrary to our voluntary fasting), hunting and chasing their prey, yet they survived.

Convergence of past and present fasting practices

Fasting existed in its natural form during the primitive times. The essence of fasting, however, evolved and was transformed as its accumulated knowledge and practice grew.

For one, we know that humans have the capacity to survive without food for days. The proof lies in the hunter-gatherer days when primitive people were forced to live without the supply of food.

The Greeks believed that medical treatment imitates nature's healing power. Observe that when you are sick, you lose the appetite to eat. It was Hippocrates who said that "to eat when you are sick is to feed your illness". You actually feel better when you abstain from food when sick. This capacity of man for self-healing is what led Philip Paracelsus to call this self-healing as the 'physician within.'

You find fasting practiced in different cultures. Mahatma Ghandi (1869 to 1948), who died at 77 through assassination, had organs like those of a 35-year-old, according to his physician. The healthy condition of Ghandi's organs was attributed to his extensive fasting.

Today, conventional medicine does not recognize natural healing. However, some physicians with a holistic outlook in medical treatments recognize the power of natural healing. Diseases exist that conventional medicine can cure, but there are diseases that fasting can prevent or reverse the damage done to cells. With more researches done on fasting and its benefits, there is hope that the conventional medicine and natural healing can converge and contribute to health.

Conventional medicine can:

- Deal with trauma
- Diagnose and treat many issues on medical and surgical emergences
- Treat bacterial infections using antibiotics
- Treat fungal and parasitic infections
- Prevent infectious diseases by immunizing affected individuals
- Diagnose medical problems that are complex

- Replace damaged knees and hips through surgery
- Do reconstructive and cosmetic surgery with good results
- Diagnose and correct deficiencies in hormones through drugs

Natural healing or fasting can:

- Treat viral infections
- Prevent or reverse the damage done by degenerative diseases
- Manage most kinds of mental illness
- Cure autoimmune disease
- Manage psychosomatic illnesses
- Reverse damage done by cancer
- Purify the body from metabolic wastes and toxins
- Stimulate cell growth
- Strengthen immune and natural defenses

Simple tips for fasting

Fasting is a safe way to heal yourself; but, there are conditions and approaches which may not be right for you. And, there are difficulties that you may experience when you fast. Some helpful tips will help you experience fasting without the inconveniences many encounter.

1. *Consult your physician*. People with health conditions, pregnant women, and people on medications should not fast. People with type 2 diabetes, those who are at risk with hyperglycemia, hypoglycemia, diabetic ketoacidosis, and dehydration should refrain from fasting.

   Stay on the safe side and consult your physician to know if you can go fasting. Your physician can also advise you on how to fast without doing harm to your health. You will know from your physician if after a prolonged fasting and toxic materials in your system have been removed, you still have the strength and resistance for the recovery and recuperation period.

2. *Experiment with different approaches*. If your purpose for fasting is to lose weight, try a modified approach. There are different approaches to fasting that you can use. Listen to how your body reacts to the approach you choose. If it

does not feel right, try a different approach.

One way to fast for weight loss is to lose weight slowly. Gradual weight loss allows you to retain a great muscle mass and keep your metabolism stimulated. An example of slow weight loss is to eliminate some foods at the start and for a few weeks.

Identify and avoid your trigger foods. Foods rich in sugar, like pastries, are difficult to eliminate. However, if you force yourself to stay away from sugar, you might rediscover the foods' natural sweetness.

3. *Adjust your exercise regimen*. If you do exercise, you might have to change the intensity of your workouts. The type of workout you do will affect your diet. For instance, if you do high-intensity workout, you may have to put this off while you are fasting. Adjust your workout to low or moderate intensity exercise. Or, instead of going to the gym you can go for a leisurely walk.

4. *Stay hydrated.* The ancient people and religious people who go on fast survived with water only. Water intake during fasting help in cleansing toxins and other impurities in your body.

   The amount of water you drink will depend on your body size, the kind of activity you do, and the environment you are in. You will be surprised that you drink less water when you fast. This reduced need for water is because you abstain from food and activities. But, you still need to drink water when fasting to keep hydrated. Observe the color of your urine. A light yellow color means you consume enough water; a darker color means your water intake is insufficient.

5. *When not fasting, plan your meals.* Regardless of what approach you use to fast, there will be breaks when you have to eat something. Your diet during fasting breaks should include balanced and nutritious foods. Remember you reduce the food intake and will therefore need nutritious foods for complete nutrition. You can have whole grains,

lean protein, vegetables, and fruits rich in healthy fats.

The gradual acceptance of fasting as a natural therapeutic remedy gives hope for its future application. Recent studies prove the existence of an invisible energy in the body that induces balance and health naturally. There are now a growing number of physicians who believe that the future medicine will pay closer attention to energy patterns and how these patterns can be enhanced to cure diseases.

Chapter 6

Ways to Start Fasting

If you decide to fast, you have a choice from a number of approaches. All types offer similar healing benefits. But, the approach you use would depend on your lifestyle, reasons for fasting, health issues you might have, and your body chemistry. You can choose any approach and will end up a winner. No one fails in fasting, for even if you do not achieve your fasting goal, you learn something of value from the experience.

Types of Fasting

1. *Intermittent Fasting*.

A layman's definition of intermittent fasting is modified abstention from food where you cycle between a period of eating and fasting. The question in this approach is when you should eat, and not what you should eat.

Intermittent fasting offers different methods to fit different people:

- <u>The 16/8 method</u> where you fast for 16 hours and eat in an 8-hour eating window. An example of an 8-hour eating window is to eat between noon and 8 in the evening only. And, within this 8-hour eating window, you can consume two, three or more meals. This method is also known as lean gains method.

  Women, though, may fast for 14 to 15 hours; they do better in shorter fast periods. This method could be difficult for people who love to eat breakfasts. It poses no problem, though, for those who skip breakfast.

- <u>Eat-Stop-Eat method</u>. In this approach, you fast for 24 hours one to two times weekly. For instance, you can plan not to eat dinner one night until dinner of the following day or from breakfast to breakfast. You then eat normally after the 24-hour fasting.

  This method can be difficult for beginners especially at the start of the plan. It will be easier if you go through this method gradually, for instance, starting with the 14 to 16-hour fasting period and move from there.

- <u>5:2 diet method</u> – In this method, you eat 500 to 600 calories for two days a week. Another name for this method is fast diet. For women, food with 500 calorie content is recommended; 600 for men.

- *Alternate-Day Fasting.* This method goes for a full fast every other day, and allows for a 500-calorie meal when not on fast. This could be difficult for beginners as you abstain from food for 24 hours. The chances are you go to bed hungry. As a beginner, you will not be able to sustain the fasting. This method is not advisable for beginners.

2. *Spiritual Fasting.*

Spiritual fasting dates back as early as the ancient times when primitive people fast to seek favor from their deities for good hunting or harvest and for spiritual purification to prove that one is deserving to offer or receive a reward from a deity.

To this day, different religions continue with the fasting tradition, though in many forms. Religious fasting is for a spiritual purpose while accepting its health benefits. The most common forms of fasting are grouped into three types: Calorie reduction (CR), alternate day fasting (ADF), and dietary restrictions (DR). Within these three types are modifications or variations in methods.

Spiritual benefits of fasting

- <u>Soul cleansing</u>. This benefit is reminiscent of the ancient fasting purpose of purification for a deity. Fasting accompanied with prayer elevates the physical self to the spiritual self where you experience a closer relationship with the Creator. Spiritual fasting accepts the close link between physical health and spiritual health. We fill ourselves with toxins with our lifestyle which leads to many kinds of illnesses. When the body is sick, the mind and spirit are sick. Therefore, as we cleanse the body with fasting, we also purify our spirit.

- <u>A renewed desire for spirituality</u>. Fasting clears your mind and becomes receptive to the inner voice which communicates with God. Hearing the inner voice talking with God gives a kind of inspiration that pushes you to a renewed spirituality.

- <u>A deeper praise</u>. Fasting gives your body a chance to rest, allowing you to focus on other matters. As you rest your body during fasting, changes happen inside you which revive your energy. The same thing happens to your spirituality. A calm body makes for a calm mind. The positive change makes us see life and everything around us as worth praising to God who created all things.

- <u>Sensitivity to God's voice</u>. The Bible gives us examples of religious people who devoted their time-serving God and being loyal to God. A purified spirit allows you to hear the inner voice and be sensitive to what it tells you. Often, this inner voice could guide you to the right path.

- <u>A new satisfaction</u>. The fasting which resulted to positive changes, both in your body and your mind, gives you new perspectives. You might realize that your usual food does not compare in value to your spiritual gain.

3. Fasting for Health.

Throughout history, people fast for recovery and recuperation from illnesses and diseases. The continued practice of fasting for health reasons to this day is proof of its effectiveness. Greek historians and philosophers believed in the benefits of fasting, and practice fasting themselves.

The Greek historian Herodotus said that the Egyptians were the healthiest people. The Egyptians fasted for three days each month by vomiting and enema to rid their bodies of toxic food.

Pythagoras and his disciples fasted for 40 days, believing that fasting clears the mind leading to an increase in perception and creativity.

The concept of fasting for health continued to the middle ages and to the present. We see physicians in recent decades advocating fasting to cure diseases:

- Friedrich Hufeland (1762 – 1836) who founded rational hygiene and used limotheraphy to cure many kinds of diseases. For him, it is best for patients not to eat anything when affected with any disease.

- De. Edward Dewey (1877) who first applied long-term fasting for curative purposes. For him, a person who lost the appetite and experienced coated tongue should not eat anything until the appetite returns. The return of appetite would indicate the functioning of the digestive system.

You will find more pioneering works in fasting and physical healing in our modern society. More researches are done on different illnesses and diseases as related to fasting. With the revived interest on fasting for health purposes, we can expect more people benefiting from fasting.

Chapter 7

What to Expect on Your First Fast

With fasting growing to be a fad and many jumping on to be "in" with the trend, it is not surprising that you would also jump in. You would think that if many are on to fasting, there must be something good in fasting.

Fasting does have health benefits. But, there is more to fasting than the common understanding of weight loss. Before you launch into a fast plan, you need to know that:

- *Fasting is not your long-term solution to weight loss*. Weight loss may be the goal for some people to go on a fast. But evident weight loss is not the achievement of a goal. One needs to continue with the diet plan to maintain the weight at the desired level. Fasting for weight loss could work for a short duration. Without planning and continued application of nutritious food choice, fasting for weight loss will fail and may be dangerous to your health.

- *You have been doing fasting every day*. You eat breakfast daily but never considered it as a form of fasting. When you sleep you *fast*, and you *break* the fast when you eat early in the morning or soon after waking up. That is how the term breakfast came about.

- *Fasting types, approaches, and methods are many*. You have a choice of fasting approach and method to suit your purpose and preference. You do not have to latch on to what you came across first. You can experiment with one type and move on to another if the previous one does not suit you.

- When you fast, follow the FAST formula:
    - **F**luids – take **fluids** always to keep you hydrated

- **A**lways – Listen to your body **always**. Your body is giving you signals about its condition
- **S**upplement - **supplement** diet plans with exercise and rest
- **T**rial - give the diet plan you choose a **trial**

What to expect on your first fast

Changes happen to your body when you fast, brought about by changes in the organs. In fasting, the metabolism changes when you take in diet foods and nutritional supplements to remove the toxins from your system. Your digestive system adjusts as it turns to stored fats for fuel energy instead of glucose.

The changes you experience in fasting depend on the type of fasting you use and the constitution of your body. You may need to consult your physician before you enter a fasting plan to know if your health is in good condition.

Stage 1:   Day 1 to 2

This is the initial stage where you abstain from food for 12 to 48 hours after your last meal. It is best to plan when and how to start fasting so you could adjust your schedule on that day with lesser activities.

What you will experience. Stage 1 is your transition stage to fasting mode, and the stage where you feel most challenged. Most beginners in fasting find the transition from normal or usual eating to fasting mode as the most difficult part. When you are hungry, you become irritable and short on patience. Expect to go through these experiences during the initial stage.

What is happening in your body. Your system draws sugar from the cells to provide the energy you need. When the sugar level goes down, you feel fatigue and hunger. To provide the necessary energy, your system turns to the stored fat in your body to use as fuel for energy. This process benefits you as you now have a supply of food to sustain you during fasting.

The benefits you get at this stage. Because of the metabolic activities going on in your body, you begin to feel the benefit in your mental and cardiovascular health. The determination you apply when fasting exercises your will power, giving you mental strength. As your BMS (Basal Metabolic Rate) lowers, you give your heart a rest, allowing it to recover from the day's stress.

Stage 2: Day 3 to 7

At this stage, more changes occur in your body, and you also begin to notice your physical appearance.

What you feel. At this stage, you start to feel the effects of ketosis. Ketosis is crucial to your fast where the body use stored fats for energy. With ketosis going on inside you, you feel less hungry and less tired. Ketosis is attracting many followers because it can allow weight loss without harming your body.

What is happening inside your body. At day 3 to 7, your body is in the fat burning mode. When not fasting, the main source of energy for the body is sugar. But, when you abstain from food, you activate the process of ketosis. In this process, your body breaks down the fats into glycerol and fatty acids. With the use of glycerol, the liver synthesizes the ketones, which is transmitted to the brain for food.

What benefits you get at stage 2. The first change in your appearance that you get to notice is your weight loss. Ketosis targets fats you don't need, like fats stored around the waist and other unlikely places. Fasting removes the accumulated toxins from your system. This cleansing system may show its effects on your skin.

Stage 3: Day 8 to 15

You notice dramatic improvements in your body, mood, and mental clarity. This is the stage where you can look forward to.

What you feel. The cleansing activity that occurred in your body in the previous stages is now having its effects. You have fully adjusted to fasting, your body purified from toxins, and your brain fed with healthy fats. Seasoned faster refer to this stage as "fasting high". The "fasting high" you feel reflects in an elevated mood, clear-mindedness, and increased energy level.

What is happening to your body. At this stage, your body is in the healing mode. Because of the cleansing process, your body has less free radicals and a reduced oxidative stress.

What benefits you get. If you reach this stage, you feel the cumulative effects of cleansing and a significant improvement of your health. When there are less free radicals in your body, you induce healthy aging and lower the risk for health complications.

Stage 4: Day 16 and onwards.

Changes due to fasting still happen during this period, but your body starts to feel the balance in your system.

What you feel. Few faster reach this stage. But, if you do, you feel balanced. At this point, you may need to consult with an expert on fasting or a health care expert who can assist you during this stage and prepare you for the completion of the fasting. You can expect no drastic changes at this stage; instead you get the feeling of being balanced. *The benefits you get*. Getting this far in your fasting activity is already an achievement. The benefits you get are satisfaction in your personal goals and growth which increases the confidence in you.

Fasting is an age-old practice which continued to the present because of the health benefits it provides. But, getting into a fasting plan needs deliberation on your part to reduce the challenges and the risks you are likely to encounter. With deliberation and a well-planned fasting experience which includes a plan on what to do after fasting, you have more chances of achieving your goal.

Chapter 8

Guide for Breaking the Fast

Some people who go fasting focus their attention on the duration of the fast, forgetting to include in the fasting plan the before and after period. Achieving your goal does not end with the completion of your fasting. Your body continues to experience change to the activities you do. Leaving from a fasting program, your body will again experience transition changes.

Have you planned for an after-fasting activity? Have you considered what happens after the completion of your fasting program?

You need to think of how to care of your body when you complete your fasting period so as not to affect your digestive system. You will lose the benefits you gained from fasting, unless you break the fast the right way.

Your body went through a series of biological changes during the fasting period. If you overeat immediately after a fast, it will be worst than overeating any time. Go slow with your food and give your system the time to adjust to its normal digestion and assimilation process. If you are not careful, eating might result to stomach cramping, vomiting, and nausea.

What to eat

What helps breaking the fast are nutritious and easy-to-digest foods, slowly adding other nutritious foods to add variety to your menu. The list of food groups below is nutritious and easy on the digestive system.

- Vegetable and fruit juices
- Raw fruits
- Bone or vegetable broths
- Unsweetened yogurt or other living, cultured dairy products
- Spinach and lettuce. You can make these vegetables appetizing by eating it

with yogurt as dressing and with a fruit juice
- Grains and beans, well-cooked
- Eggs and nuts
- Non-cultured milk products
- Lean meats

Food you should not eat:
- Fatty meat
- White flour and products with white flour
- Fried foods, especially those fried with unhealthy fatty oil
- White rice, pasty, and white bread
- Carbonated beverages including diet soda
- Chemical sugar substitutes and refined sugar
- Food with shortening and margarine
- Food with animal fat and high fat products

Guides in eating after a fast

1) Listen to the reaction or signals your body sends when you eat new foods. Watch for negative reactions from your body, like mild allergy. Body signals from your body could tell you if you

have gone far with your food. Be sensitive to what you feel, like the sensation of fullness. When you feel full, stop eating. When you make listening to your body a practice, you will be alerted to the state of your body.

2) Begin with small meals consumed frequently. You could start with 2 hours and progress into larger meals with longer time in between. This meal progression will allow your digestive system to adjust until it gets to its normal routine, like three meals a day with in between snacks.

3) Chew foods well to help your digestive system. Chewing food is a good habit to cultivate. Do not hurry with your meals as this will also affect your digestive system.

4) Try to include live enzymes and good bacteria to your system. Include raw foods and good bacteria in your meals.

How to determine if you succeed in your fasting goal

You will know if you succeed in your fasting if you see the following indicators:

- You achieve your goal in fasting
- You are able to complete the duration of your fast. Many stopped at some point in their fasting, usually towards the end of the fasting duration.
- You get the maximum healing gains from your fasting
- You successfully transitioned in and out of the fasting program
- You improved your dietary habits and your lifestyle after the fast
- You are able to maintain your weight loss after the program

How to achieve success in fasting

If you are a beginner in fasting, you will have more chances of success if you prepare and plan for fasting.

1) *Identify your objectives for fasting*. Are you clear with why you want to fast? You need to be clear with your objective

as this serves as your anchor during the duration of the fast. Your objective will spur you on, especially when you feel you are wavering in your intent.
.

2) *Be in the right frame of mind* before starting your fast. It helps to be in the right state of mind with the following:
   - Get hold of fasting resources and immerse yourself in them.
   - Read fasting logs of others, particularly those seasoned faster.
   - Satisfy yourself with your favorite food before fasting. This will stop your craving for such food once you are into fasting.

3) *Choose a length of fasting you think you can manage*. You get more benefits the longer you stay in fasting mode. The initial stage introduces you to fasting and allows for a slow transition to make the adjustment easy for you. Healing begins in the fourth day when ketosis begins. Match the length of your fasting with your objective.

4) *Don't psych yourself out*. Most people who fail in their fasting allow mental

barriers that prevent them from persevering. At the slightest challenge encountered, they say "I can't do this", "This fasting is not for me", "I need food or I get a headache."

Mental barriers are more successful in stopping you from fasting than the physical barriers. However, the only person who can correct this is you. Turn these negative thoughts into positive ones and commit to your objectives. Turn to fasting resources to get inspiration and motivation.

5) *You don't have to announce your fast.* You never know how people would react to any information you send out. If mental and physical barriers don't affect you, negative reactions from others might just be successful. And you fail with your fasting objective even before you begin.

You will encounter many challenges in fasting, like fatigue, headaches, lethargy, and perhaps hunger pains. If you add to the list friends and family members who are not amenable to fasting as an alternative therapy, their negative reactions might influence you. At the weakened state you are in, you might just give in to their negative suggestions.

6) *Deal with your emotions while on fasting*. Expect to go through different emotions when you fast. You are likely to feel sadness, anger, irritation, self-hate, guilt, and cravings to name a few. Experiencing these emotions happen with longer periods of fasting. Work through these emotions; you can block them out, you can sleep, or you can face your emotions and work through them. How you choose to deal with your emotions is not important; what matters is the closure.

You can work through your emotions by:

- o Identifying the emotion. If you are experiencing multiple emotions, pick one to work on and move to the next once you achieved your closure.

- o Understand where the emotion is coming from. For instance, if you feel anger, try to understand why you feel angry and what is making you angry.
  - o Understand the context which brought out the emotion.
  - o Get closure once you have identified and understood the emotion.

7) *Go for a maximum bed rest*. Sleep is important to you. This is the time when the cells in your body go to work to repair and recycle damaged cells without any intrusion from your activities. The schedule which you prepare for fasting is also intended for this purpose, to give your body the maximum rest it needs.

8) *Commit to your post-fast plan.* Commitment to your post-fast plan will determine the success of your fasting.

There is a reason for the increasing popularity of fasting. It not only heals you physically, but purifies your body, mind and spirit. Fasting because it is fashionable will fail. But, there is no need for you to fail in your desire to fast. You have it in you to get hold of the resources to make your fasting successful.

Conclusion

Thank you again for downloading this book!

To be blunt, it is not easy to fast and you may only see some results after a couple of weeks. You will gain increased energy level as well as fit and healthy body. It is also possible that you may need to change the type of intermittent fasting that you follow. If you have followed my suggestion regarding acclimation, you should have chosen the most suitable type of intermittent fasting.

To tell you the truth, it took me some time before I was able to find the most suitable type of fasting that I truly prefer. I wrote about acclimation because I went through the process of finding the most suitable one for me the hard way. It came to a point where I almost gave up and I sure am glad that I never did. If I have given up early on, I won't be able to experience all the wonderful benefits that I enjoy today.

I want you to experience the amazing things that changed my life for good. I hope that this book will be able to help you change your life for the better.

If you enjoyed this book, please take the time to share your thoughts and post a review on Amazon. It'd be greatly appreciated!

Thank you and good luck!